Filling the FOLDS of Aging

Aging may be inevitable, but the rate of aging is not. Chronological age has little bearing on biological age. The number of candles on your birthday cake merely serves as a marker of time not your health.

Protein contains amino acids called L-lysine and L-proline, which are very important in the creation of collagen in your body. Collagen gives structure to your skin's tissues. As you get older, your collagen breaks down, which may lead to wrinkles. So eating a high-protein diet fortifies your collagen levels and therefore makes your skin thicker and less prone to wrinkles.

The building blocks that make up all proteins, including collagen, are called **amino acids**. If you lack the amino acids that combine to form collagen, your body's cells can't produce enough of it.

I0445879

Collagen is a type of protein, and works with keratin to provide the skin with strength, smoothness, elasticity and resilience. The skin and other parts of the body produce it. When you are young, you have an abundance of collagen in your body, which is why young children have such lovely shiny hair and smooth skin. It is referred to, as the cement, which holds everything together. As you age collagen production declines and weakening of the skin occurs, this is when skin wrinkles, necks become saggy, lines form around eyes and mouth.

The skin is made up of three layers, epidermis, dermis and hypodermis. The second layer of the skin (dermis) is where the protein collagen is found. Collagen molecules are bundled together throughout the dermis.

Threonine is an essential amino acid for collagen production. An essential amino acid is one your body cannot make, so you have to get it from food or dietary supplements. You can get threonine from foods such as lentils, peanuts, eggs, milk, pork, beef and chicken. If you prefer a vegetarian diet, you can also get threonine from soybeans, chickpeas, hummus, snap beans and asparagus. Everything from a chicken dinner to a mid-day peanut snack may provide a benefit to your skin.

Another amino acid that aids in collagen production is **proline**. Unlike threonine, proline is a nonessential amino acid; nonessential amino acids are ones that either the body or other essential amino acids can produce. You can also help your body by eating foods high in proline, such as gelatin, soy, milk, cheese, beef and cabbage. And as we mentioned before, vitamin C works along with proline to promote collagen production. Foods such as oranges, lemons and limes contain vitamin C.

Two benefits of a high-protein diet are healthy skin and increased muscle mass. Protein is full of amino acids that create collagen in your body, a substance that thickens your skin and leaves it looking clearer. Protein is also the only food group that makes your muscles grow, because it stimulates the production of cells in your muscles.

We are the some of our life experiences.
We have had decades to develop and maintain habits that have an impact on our health, both negatively and positively.
Aging is universal, but each of us experiences it in different ways.

The complexities of getting older make it difficult to pinpoint why one person ages well while another looks and acts older than her years. If your father died young of a heart attack and your mother had breast cancer, you may be genetically predisposed to those diseases.

Genes are powerful predictors of health and longevity, as well as disease and death, but they're only a part of the story. If your parents and grandparents lived well into their nineties, chances are you will too; but not if you abuse your body along the way.

There is no question that a healthy lifestyle is your weapon against the genes you've been dealt. Healthy living delays many of the body changes that aging brings. It's never too late to start on the road to better health. Eating a nutritious diet goes a long way toward insuring good health.

Physiological changes occur slowly over time in all body systems. The changes are influences by life events, illnesses, genetic traits, socioeconomic factors, and nutrition.

People of all ages need more than 40 nutrients to stay healthy. With age, it becomes more important that diets contain enough calcium, fiber, iron, protein, and the Vitamins A, C, D and folic acid.

Cells, the most basic body unit, are at the center of any discussion about aging. You have trillions of cells, and over time, cell death outpaces cell production, leaving us with fewer cells. As a result, we are less capable of repairing wear and tear on the body, and our immune system is compromised. Though cell death is the basis for understanding the aging process, it is not the only factor.

It is unquestionably true that a significant number of problems faced by people over the age of 60 may also be attributable to nutritional deficiencies. Many elderly people have malabsorption problems, in which the nutrients in food are not properly absorbed from the gastrointestinal tract. In addition, as we age, our bodies do not assimilate nutrients as well as they once did. At the same time, as the body ages, its systems slow down and become less efficient, so the correct nutrients are more important than ever for the support, repair, and regeneration of the cells. There are many disorders associated with an inability to absorb nutrients successfully.

One can have vitality and a zest for living at any age. You should not assume that pain and illness are inevitable parts of aging. You can feel better at 60 than you did at 30 by making healthy changes in your diet and lifestyle.

Adding the right supplements should give you the added power needed to boost immunity and prevent or cure most disorders – not to mention making you able to work or play longer than people much younger than you are. Looking youthful for your age in an added bonus. It takes years for these problems to develop, so it usually takes some time to resolve them as well. There are no silver bullets or magic potions, only the simple fact that if you give your body the correct fuel; it will perform for you and ward off illness.

Many older people become deficient in B12 because they do not produce adequate amounts of stomach acid for proper digestion. This creates a perfect environment for the overgrowth of certain bacteria that steal whatever Vitamin B12 is extracted from protein in the digestive tract. Vitamin B12 deficiency is a particular problem. A lack of Vitamin B12 can lead to the development of neurological symptoms ranging from tingling sensations, inability to coordinate muscular movements, weakened limbs, and lack of balance, to memory loss, mood changes, disorientation, and psychiatric disorders. Symptoms of Vitamin B12 deficiency can easily be misinterpreted as signs of **senility**.

Drugs used to control diseases such as hypertension or heart disease can alter the need for electrolytes, sodium and potassium. Even though absorption and utilization of some vitamins and minerals becomes less effective with age, higher intakes do not appear to be necessary.

Growing older is inevitable; however, we can try to slow the aging process and prolong our lives by taking measures to promote continuous cell division. If science could keep cells from dying and doing bodily harm, the aging process could conceivably be suspended.
Aging in not an illness, but it does make the body more vulnerable to disease. There are many theories on aging and its causes.

Benjamin Franklin one said, "We get old too soon and wise too late."
Applying a little wisdom may keep you from aging before your time.
Only 5-20 percent of the aging process has to do with our genes; the rest has to do with how we treat our bodies.

Nutrition can be a factor in a lot of bodily changes. The slowing of the normal action of the digestive tract plus general changes have the most direct effect on nutrition. Digestive secretions diminish markedly, although enzymes remain adequate. Adequate dietary fiber, as opposed to increased use of laxatives, will maintain regular bowel function and not interfere with the digestion and absorption of nutrients, as occurs with laxative use of abuse. The challenge for the elderly is to meet the same nutrient needs as when they were younger, yet consume fewer calories.

Protein absorption may decrease as we age, and our bodies may take less protein.

Adequate fiber, altogether with adequate fluid, helps maintain normal bowel function. Fiber also is thought to decrease risk of intestinal inflammation. Vegetables, fruits, grain products, cereals, seeds, legumes, and nuts are all sources of dietary fiber.

Iron and calcium intake sometimes appears to be low in many elderly. To

improve absorption of iron, include
vitamin C-rich fruits and vegetables.
Zinc can be related to specific diseases
in the elderly. It can also be a factor
with vitamin K in wound healing. Zinc
improves taste acuity in people where
stores are low. If you eat meats, eggs,
and seafood, zinc intake should be
adequate.

Zinc along with vitamin C and E, and
the phytochemicals lutein, zeaxanthin
and beta-carotene may help prevent or
slow the onset of age-related macular
(eye) degeneration. The best way to
obtain these nutrients is to consume at
least five servings of fruits and
vegetables, especially dark green,
orange, and yellow ones. Good choices
include kale, spinach, broccoli, peas,
oranges, and cantaloupes. Consult your
doctor to see if a supplement may also
be necessary.

Vitamin E may have a potential role in
the prevention of Alzheimer's disease.
Research has shown that eating foods
with vitamin E, like whole grains, nuts,

and seeds, may help reduce the risk of Alzheimer's disease.

Low levels of vitamin B12 have been associated with memory loss and linked to age-related hearing loss in older adults. Folate, which is related to vitamin B12 metabolism in the body, may actually improve hearing. If vitamin B12 levels are not adequate, high folate levels may be a health concern. As we age, the amount of the chemical in the body, needed to absorb vitamin B12 decreases. To avoid deficiency, older adults are advised to eat foods rich in vitamin B12 regularly, including meat, poultry, fish, eggs, and dairy foods.

Of all nutrients, **Water is the most important, serving many essential functions.**

Adequate water intake reduces stress on kidney function, which tends to decline with age. Adequate fluid intake also eases constipation. With the aging process, the ability to detect thirst declines; so do not wait to drink water until you are thirsty. Drink plenty of water, juice, milk, and coffee and tea to stay hydrated. Drink the equivalent to five to eight glasses everyday. It may be helpful to use a cup or water bottle, which has calibrated measurements on it, in order to keep track of how much you drink. Carry it with you throughout your home or wherever you go during the day.

There are 4 possible reasons, which are thought to be dangerous processes that age our bodies and are triggered by the food we eat and the lifestyles we lead.

Free Radicals, Inflammation, Sugar, and Stress.

Free radicals: Similar to the way rust attacks a car, free radicals – chemically unstable molecules – attack our cells and damage our DNA, a process that many experts believe accelerates aging. Free radicals are also known to increase the risk of cancer. You can't, unfortunately, completely avoid these molecules – they're present in the air you breathe – but you can limit your exposure to them by avoiding things like cigarettes, trans fats (partially hydrogenated oils which have been banned from many foods), excess sun exposure, charred meats, and other sources. Organic fruits and vegetables limit your exposure to pesticides and herbicides, which also contain the harmful molecules. If you can't afford to go completely organic, try to at least buy the following foods organically: peaches, apples, blueberries, bell peppers, celery, nectarines, strawberries, cherries, imported grapes, spinach, kale, and potatoes. Fruits and vegetables are also chock full of antioxidants, which are thought to neutralize free radicals, so you should still aim to get five servings a day, organic or not. Those with the highest amount of antioxidants include prunes, raisins, blueberries, blackberries, and kale.

Inflammation: Some aging factors are beyond our control, but one of the **biggest** – inflammation – needn't be. Here's how you can extinguish the flames of chronic inflammation before they ignite.

Under ordinary circumstances, inflammation is a healthy process that comes to the body's aid when it's injured. For instance, if you cut your finger while making dinner, the body's inflammatory response sends in an army of white blood cells to the scene. These cellular mercenaries destroy lurking bacteria while mending any ragged tissue. By the time you can see and feel physical signs of inflammation – heat, soreness and swelling – the cut is probably well on its way to healing.

Unfortunately, inflammation isn't always so exact. Like a houseguest who overstays his welcome, inflammation sometimes hangs around too long and refuses to leave. Aging is one of the biggest risk factors for inflammation, since, as we age, our bodies are less able to disarm the inflammatory process. A genetic predisposition, high blood pressure or even smoking can also fuel the flames. When the inflammation switch refuses to turn off, the body operates as if it is always under attack. White blood cells flood the system for weeks, months and even years.

The problem is that the immune system can't handle the constant demand. When the immune system becomes drained, the body then has difficulty warding off other illnesses. For instance, viruses, bacterial infections, even cancer cells that are normally destroyed by a healthy immune system can now slip under the body's radar. Ultimately, the immune system may even turn against the body itself – the consequences of which are quite serious: Lupus, Graves' disease, Crohn's disease and fibromyalgia are all autoimmune disorders that come about when the body is assaulted by its own defenses.

Normally part of a healthy immune response to foreign invaders, inflammation is now considered to be a major player in many diseases of aging including cancer, diabetes, heart disease, and Alzheimer's – that is, when it becomes chronic. This happens when the immune system begins targeting healthy cells and tissues for attack.
Inflammation can operate in stealth mode for years. When symptoms do finally become apparent, it's usually in these forms, as mentioned earlier, of diabetes, osteoarthritis or other inflammation-related diseases.

For a way to reduce inflammation in the body, try to follow a Mediterranean style diet based on whole grains, fatty fish like salmon and tuna, fruits, vegetables, and monounsaturated fats (nuts, avocados, and olives) with little meat.

Other great anti-inflammatory foods include" spices like turmeric, chocolate (the really dark kind that has 70 percent or higher cacao content), and red wine, which contain the anti-aging chemical resveratrol. However, resveratrol may prove more useful as a supplement, since you would have to drink more than 100 bottles of wine a day to make any real impact on the aging process.

Exercise is another great way to lower inflammation by boosting anti-inflammatory chemicals and helping you avoid weight gain through the years.
Having too much belly fay, defined as a waist measurement of more than 35 inches for a woman and 40 inches for a man, means you probably have high inflammation, since abdominal fat produces inflammatory chemicals.
Aim for a moderate amount of steady exercise like brisk walking, swimming, or biking for 30 to 45 minutes five days a week. But don't overdo it to the point of soreness and extreme fatigue, since

too much exercise can actually increase inflammation.

Most foods either rev up inflammation or tamp it down. A diet high in trans-fatty acids, carbohydrates and sugar drives the body to create inflammatory chemicals. On the flip side, a diet heavy on vegetables, lean meats, whole grains and omega-3 fatty acids puts the brakes on the inflammatory process.

Early humans consumed an excellent balance of pro-inflammatory fats (mainly omega-6s) and anti-inflammatory fats (such as omega-3s and -9s). People today, however, often chow down on 30 times more bad fats than good. The typical American diet is priming people for inflammation.

What you eat helps determine how much inflammation you produce. Certain foods promote it, while others are inflammation-fighting superstars.

Use...

- **Omega-3 fats**: These are among the most potent anti-inflammatory foods. Best sources are fatty fish like salmon and tuna, walnuts and other nuts, flaxseed, and canola oil.
- **Colorful produce**: Red onions, tomatoes, broccoli, red grapes, berries, and oranges all are packed with chemicals called flavonoids that have anti-inflammatory properties.
- **Herbs and spices**: Ginger and turmeric, either dried or fresh, are among the most healthful spices. For herbs, sprinkle on some fresh rosemary.
- **Chocolate and wine**: Red wine has anti-inflammatory chemicals like resveratrol. Dark chocolate – look for 70 percent or higher cacao – protects against inflammation.

Cut back on…

- **Omega-6 fats**: They trigger the body to produce pro-inflammatory chemicals. Oils in omega-6 fats include corn, safflower, and vegetable oils; mayonnaise, and many salad dressings.
- **Trans fats**: They're disappearing from packaged foods as more and more research shows they drive inflammation. And now they're on nutrition labels, so they're easier to avoid.
- **Rancid fats**: Don't heat oil to the point that it's smoking, since that oxidizes fats and turns them into inflammation boosters. Also, avoid old peanut butter and that chocolate bar stashed away for years in your pantry.
- **White starches**: Flour, sugar, white rice, and instant mashed potatoes, for example, all cause quick spikes in blood sugar

levels, causing the production of advanced glycation end products that spur inflammation.
- **Animal fats**: Foods high in this fat – egg yolks, red meat, poultry skin, and whole-milk dairy products – also contain high amounts of arachidonic acid, a molecule used by the body to create inflammation.
- **Excess alcohol**: Avoid drinking more than one or two alcoholic beverages a day; too much alcohol can cause changes in the intestinal lining, allowing bacteria to pass through into the bloodstream, triggering inflammation.

Glycation: This is a fancy word for too much sugar, or rather, what happens when the sugar mixes with proteins and fats to form molecules that promote aging. Advanced glycation en products, or AGEs, are thought to accelerate the aging process by churning out free radicals and promoting inflammation. They form when you caramelize onions in a frying pan, for example, or mix a little sugar in with that omelet you're cooking. To avoid AGEs, turn down the heat when you cook. The browning effect that occurs when you stir-fry vegetables at high heat or blacken chicken in a frying pan causes these molecules to form, especially if you're adding sugar to the mix. Limiting your intake of sugar-filled foods in general will also help, since excess sugar often binds to protein in your body to form AGEs. Aside from increasing your risk of heart disease, AGEs appear to play a role in diabetes by causing blood to become sticky and hampering its ability to flow smoothly through capillaries and into the extremities and vital organs like the kidneys and eyes. Glycation is like putting sugar in your gas tank, it gums up the works.

We all know that when it comes to our bodies, sugar is a sly villain—falling prey to its siren song will give our taste buds a hit of pleasure before wreaking havoc everywhere else. But there probably aren't many of us who worry that eating it might also cause wrinkles—and that's not a sweet story either.

The proteins in skin most prone to glycation are the same ones that make a youthful complexion so plump and springy—collagen and elastin. When those proteins hook up with renegade sugars, they become discolored, weak, and less supple; this shows up on the skin's surface as wrinkles, sagginess, and a loss of radiance.

Diet and lifestyle choices can affect how quickly the effects of glycation can be seen on the skin.

Stress: Damage to DNA is the culprit behind wrinkles, gray hair, and diseases that can shorten our lifespan.

Being under pressure initiates the release of a variety of stress hormones that make your pulse race and cause your blood pressure to rise. But the hormone cortisol, released to lessen these effects, actually creates problems when it remains chronically elevated. It can also lead to the accumulation of belly fat, causing inflammation and insulin resistance. Practicing relaxation techniques like meditation or yoga may help manage stress. Getting too little sleep is akin to feeling too much stress in terms of your body's increases production of cortisol, so make sure to aim for 7-8 hours a night.

There's quite a bit of hype out there about toxins these days. You may hear reports about how toxic buildups in the body can lead to cellulite, constipation, fatigue, and even autoimmune disease. Any number of horrible illnesses and health conditions has been attributed to toxins of late. Even more publicity is swirling about the need to detoxify, cleanse, or purify your body. The current levels of pollution, pesticides, contaminants and artificial substances in processed foods may affect your body and all its systems. Especially in high doses, toxins have the ability to speed up the **aging process**, disrupt hormones, suppress your immune system, mangle your memory, and can sometimes even lead to cancer.

Exposure to environmental toxins has been pinpointed as one of the causes of aging. When regularly exposed to environmental toxins – which we all are – your body can get bogged down with chronic oxidative stress, and free radicals may go on a rampage. Most organ systems can be harmed, but it is the brain that is perhaps most vulnerable. Oxidative stress caused by toxins could be a major cause of Alzheimer's disease, other types of dementia, and Parkinson's disease.

The human body is the best detoxification system in the world. You were born fully equipped with a very powerful waste management system. When it's functioning properly, you are naturally able to rid yourself of most of the toxins you encounter as each system can adequately dump its waste into the urinary and digestive systems, which then release them out of your body. Your skin also acts as a way for your body to flush out waste—in the form of sweat! So, to help your body filter and release toxins before they accumulate, it is important to stay healthy and keep all of your systems functioning properly.

Wrinkles are creases, folds or ridges in the skin. Most commonly, wrinkles appear, as we get older. However, they may develop after our skin has been immersed in water for a long time. The first wrinkles to appear on our face tend to occur as a result of facial expressions. Sun damage, smoking, dehydration, some medications, as well as a number of other factors may also cause wrinkles to develop.

Wrinkles form when the skin thins and loses its elasticity. As long as the skin is supple, any creasing of the skin disappears as soon as you stop making the expression that caused it. But skin that has lost its suppleness retains the lines formed by smiling or frowning, for instance, even after you have assumed a more neutral expression. Over time, these lines deepen into wrinkles.

Some amount of wrinkling is a result of aging and is probably inevitable; no matter what you do, you will develop some lines if you simply live long enough.

Whether you're 35 and just beginning to see the first signs of aging, or 55 with skin that isn't exactly keeping your birthday a secret, seeking ways to reduce wrinkles is probably on your agenda.

Wrinkles may be an inevitable part of aging, but that doesn't mean fighting them is useless. Protecting your skin from exposure to ultraviolet radiation is the most significant thing you can do to prevent wrinkles, sagging, and discoloration. And some people try invasive techniques, such as chemical peels, Botox, dermal fillers, or surgery. But those efforts are all done from the outside. What is protecting your skin from the inside?

What you eat or don't eat has a definite effect on the health of your skin. As your body's outermost barrier and largest organ, your skin is continuously exposed to various sources of stress, including many environmental factors.

So, although a new diet won't clear away all your wrinkles or halt skin aging, nutrition can make a huge difference not only in how you look but also in how you feel.

It may not be a sure cure for crow's feet, brow furrows, or laugh lines, but improving a few food and behavior choices could help your skin. Although studies specific to wrinkle prevention are currently limited, a host of other studies reveal that the same vitamins and nutrients that may protect your skin also are beneficial to the health of your eyes, teeth, nails, bones, and circulatory system. So if a more youthful appearance overall is what you're after, then skin is only part of the equation. Eating a diverse diet with plenty of fruit and vegetables can make your Real Age younger and can bring out a healthier and younger-looking you.

The Skin is the largest organ in the body – about 20 square feet – and the most vulnerable organ in the body. It's exposed to both oxidizing effects of UV radiation from the sun and the oxidizing effects of oxygen in the air, and years of oxidant stress can take a toll. As we age, our skin becomes thinner, more easily damaged, loses volume and elasticity, and can sag and wrinkle. So what can we do about it?

The Do's and Don'ts of Wrinkles:

Avoid the sun: It's the No. 1 cause of wrinkles, with dozens of studies documenting the impact.

Wear sunscreen: If you must go out in the sun, wear sunscreen. It will protect you from skin cancer, and help prevent wrinkles at the same time.

Don't smoke: Cigarette smoke ages skin – mostly by releasing an enzyme that breaks down collagen and elastin, important components of the skin.

Get adequate sleep: When you don't get enough sleep, the body produces excess cortisol, a hormone that breaks down skin cells. Get enough rest and you'll produce more HGH (Human Growth Hormone – Hormone of youth), which helps the skin remain thick, more "elastic", and less likely to wrinkle.

Sleep on your back: Sleeping in certain positions night after night leads to "sleep lines" – wrinkles that become etched into the surface of the skin and don't disappear once you are up. Sleeping on your side increases wrinkles on cheeks and chin, while sleeping face down gives you a furrowed brow. To reduce wrinkle formation, sleep on your back.

Don't squint – get reading glasses: Any repetitive facial movement – like squinting – overworked facial muscles, forming a groove beneath the skin's surface. This groove eventually becomes a wrinkle. Also important: wear sunglasses. It will protect skin around the eyes from sun damage – and further keep you from squinting.

Eat more fish – particularly salmon: Not only is salmon (along with other cold water fish) a great source of protein – one of the building blocks of great skin – it's also an awesome source of an essential fatty acid known as omega-3. Essential fatty acids help nourish skin and keep it plump and youthful, helping to reduce wrinkles.

Eat more soy: Certain properties of (fermented) soy may help protect or heal some of the sun's photoaging damage. Soy-based supplement (other ingredients including fish protein and extracts for white tea, grapeseed, and tomato, as well as several vitamins) improved skin's structure and firmness after just six months of use.

Trade coffee for cocoa: Cocoa containing high levels of two dietary flavanols (epicatechin and catechin) protected the skin from sun damage, improved circulation to skin cells, affected hydration, and made the skin look and feel smoother.

Eat more fruits and vegetables: The key is their antioxidant compound. These compounds fight damage caused by free radicals (unstable molecules that damage cells), which in turn help skin look younger and more radiant, and protects against some effects of photoaging.

Use moisturizer: Women, especially, are so concerned with antiaging products they often overlook the power of a simple moisturizer. Skin that is moist simply looks better, so lines and creases are far less noticeable.

Don't over wash your face: Tap water strips skin of its natural barrier oils and moisture that protects against wrinkles.

Wash them off too often, and you wash away protection. Moreover, unless your soap contains moisturizers, you should use a cleanser instead.

The RDI is used to determine the **Daily Value** (**DV**) of foods, which is printed on nutrition facts labels in the United States and Canada, which is regulated by the Food and Drug Administration (FDA).

The USDA (**United States Department of Agriculture**), also known as the **Agriculture Department**, is responsible for developing and executing federal government policy on farming, agriculture, forestry, and food.

Consult with your physician or doctor before starting or stopping a nutritional or fitness program or medications.

Foods to Fight Aging

Experts suspect that vitamin A, C, and E and the minerals zinc and selenium may keep wrinkles at bay by reducing the amount of potentially damaging free radicals produced by skin cells. And carotenoid-rich fruit and veggies such as cantaloupe, apricots, carrots, sweet potatoes, and spinach may also boost your skin's health. Choose fruits and vegetables that have deep green, yellow, orange, and red hues. The intense color is the calling card of carotenoids.

Minimize your intake of simple or high glycemic index carbohydrates, such as enriched bread or flour products, processed and refined foods, candy, and soft drinks. These are often low in nutrients and high in sugar. Instead choose complex or low glycemic index carbs, such as legumes and whole grain breads and cereals.

Healthy Food choices for your Skin

Vitamin A
- Spinach, leaf lettuce, carrots, squash, sweet potatoes
- Papayas, mangoes, cantaloupe
- Low-fat milk, eggs

Vitamin C
- Red bell peppers, broccoli
- Peaches, oranges, papayas, kiwi

Vitamin E
- Nuts and seeds

Zinc and Selenium
- Fortified whole-grain cereals
- Eggs, low-fat milk

The **USDA** recommends your diet be made up of 18 percent protein. This means you will only eat 91 g of protein per day in a typical diet. However, on a high-protein diet you get 30 to 50 percent of your daily calorie needs from protein, so you are eating at least 1 g of protein for every pound of body weight.

Lean meats and fish are the best sources of protein for your body and skin, because they are high in protein but also low in saturated fat. Burgers, New York strip steaks and hot dogs give you protein, but their high fat content increases your cholesterol levels. This stops blood from reaching your muscles and cells and will lead to deceased muscle mass and blotchy skin. Instead, choose boneless, skinless chicken or turkey, flank steak, extra-lean pork, or fish, such as salmon or mackerel.

Other sources of protein include egg whites, lentils, beans, peas, nuts, cheese, soymilk and whole wheat cereals. Vegetarians must be very disciplined to make sure they get enough dietary protein, but if you eat meat, you should get some of your daily protein quota from vegetarian sources, because this will lower your cholesterol.

Bibliography

http://www.ext.colostate.edu
http://www.webmd.com
http://www.sharecare.com
http://smartskincare.com
http://www.howstuffworks.com
http://health.usnews.com
http://www.experience life.com
http://www.medicalnewstoday.com
http://www.drmikediet.com